INTERMITTENT FASTING

INTERMITTENT FASTING

My Ebook Publishing House
Bucharest, 2018

CONTENTS

INTRODUCTION

I want to thank and congratulate you for purchasing this book – Intermittent Fasting

Intermittent Fasting is a phenomenon that is currently one of the world's most famous health and fitness trends. It involves a process of following alternating cycles of fasting and eating.

This book contains proven steps and strategies on how to fast intermittently for weight loss and also examines the concept of clean eating.

By reading it, you will learn practical and time-proven arts and practices that if religiously followed, will create a youthful, vibrant, exuberant, radiant and entirely different you!

aim is usually for calorie confinement which aids weight loss.

Somehow, intermittent fasting can be said to be the old mystery of sound health. It is tagged old-fashioned because it has been around ever since the very existence of humanity. I have also labeled a mystery since this strong predisposition has been practically overlooked.

So can intermittent fasting be said to a form of starvation or an excuse for malnourishment?

No. intermittent fasting varies from starvation in one crucial way – you control your craving. Starvation on the hand is the routine lack of food. It can neither be managed nor controlled which invariably leads to malnourishment. This is a different thing entirely from fasting, which happens to be the willful withholding of food and other nourishment for profound, wellbeing, or a different reason entirely.

In the case of fasting, food is readily accessible, but you simply don't want to eat it. This might include working with a particular timeframe, which could be a couple of hours in a day or a longer timeframe. The thing about fasting is that you decide when to start and when to stop at your convenience owning to reasons best known to you.

Conversely, Intermittent fasting cannot be said to be an eating routine. Instead, it involves consuming fewer calories nutrition design.

On a lighter note, some individuals are trying to refining this kind of dietary mediation as it seems this individual now understand the enormous advantages intermittent fasting conveys if appropriately done such as assisting weight loss, expanded vitality, decreasing the possibility of having type 2 diabetes and lots more. Additionally, it will help spare cash and other valuable resources.

As of late, intermittent fasting has turned out to be progressively recognized with sportspeople, and individuals trying to stay fit or enhance their wellbeing.

In simpler terms, intermittent fasting implies merely the need to expend calories diet amid a particular timeframe and pick not to eat nourishment for a more significant window of time.

Intermittent fasting can be categorized into two classifications:

- Whole day fasting and
- Time-restricted feeding (TRF)

Talking about entire day fasting, then we will be referring to fasting for a full day. The strictest shape would be Alternate day fasting. This is usually a follow-up for a complete 24-hours of the nonfasting period.

Time-restricted feeding on its part includes eating just in the middle of specific hours daily. A typical example of TRF includes fasting for about 16 hours daily and eating in-between the rest of the 8 hours, and following a similar timetable righteously daily.

There are lots of approaches that can be expended amid fasting timeframes. While some will stick to water, some may consider taking a cup of coffee or tea without sugar or milk; some others will prefer drinks with zero calories with designed sweeteners while some will instead not go for anything. However, others would go for "adjustable fasting" with constrained caloric intake during their fasting periods instead of going for none by any means.

Certain facts on intermittent fasting

- There is banter among scientists and other health researchers about the best strategy for intermittent fasting.
- Intermittent fasting might be more compelling for excessive weight loss than muscle building.

- Fasting may impact growth faction, and additionally aid response to treatment of disease.
- Studies have further proven that individuals following an intermittent fasting design can likewise stick to a modified cardiovascular activity.

CHAPTER TWO

THE MOST EFFECTIVE WAY OF DOING INTERMITTENT FASTING

As earlier stated, intermittent fasting has been around the human race for a long time, and a few distinct techniques have been utilized.

Every one of the methods used has been in one way or the other included a periodic distinction between "eating and fasting periods." Amid the fasting period, it is expected that you eat little or nothing at all by any stretch of the imagination.

However, certain strategies are primarily recognized among people who do intermittent fasting. These include;

The 16/8 Strategy: often referred to as Leangains strategy- This strategy is targeted toward skipping breakfasts and limiting the daily eating period to nothing less than 8 hours per day, which invariably means fasting" for 16 hours in between.

The 5:2 eating regimens: This strategy focuses more on some certain days in the week, probably the last two days of the week, where you are expected to eat 500-600 calories. After then, you can normally eat for the remaining five days.

Eat-Stop-Eat: This strategy is better known as the whole-day fasting as it includes fasting for complete 24 hours, for a whole seven days. For instance, should you have dinner now, then you'll have to skip food until the following day dinner time before eating anything, thus, completing the whole of 24 hrs?

Recently, a survey assessing intermittent fasting found that overweight or corpulent people with diabetes (the type diabetes) who fast on whole or alternate days are at a more significant advantage to reduce obesity and similarly to encounter upgraded cardiovascular medical edges.

The remedial capability of intermittent fasting stayed notwithstanding when included in the calorie consumption daily which doesn't change anything somewhat decreased marginally.

Neurological sicknesses

Intermittent fasting may likewise affect insight. In a test carried out on rodents with qualities for Alzheimer's ailment, intermittent fasting enhanced execution on measures of subjective decay related to maturing.

Glucose

Studies have proven that intermittent fasting enhances affectability of insulin better than other diet control plans, although these investigations have not thoroughly tested with a concrete standpoint. Medical experts globally have also confirmed that intermittent fasting and other dieting modules prompt practically identical reductions in the body system hemoglobin A1c

Are there any potential dangers associated with intermittent fasting?

Everything has pros and cons, and so does intermittent fasting. The truth is, intermittent fasting isn't healthy for everybody. Certain individuals aren't advised to take on intermittent fasting, some of them include:

- Underweight Individuals
- People with Dietary issues
- Type 1 diabetes patients
- Drug-induced Type 2 diabetes patients
- Pregnant women
- Individuals just recovering from surgical sessions
- Depressed individuals
- Sick people

Disadvantages of intermittent fasting

- Changes in temperament
- Odd appetite
- Low dynamism
- Obsessive considerations about nourishment
- Voraciously consuming foodways

In summary, intermittent fasting is a good eating regimen, but, it does have its pros and cons!!!

Intermittent fasting can be taken as a module for staying in shape for people in a perfect world with stable and rational association with food which needs to keep fit without exercising much and consuming fewer calories.

How then is intermittent fasting IF comparable with Grazing?

Productive nourishment designs, regardless of whether they utilize littler, more successive meals or bigger, less continuous suppers all offer a couple of similar features.

These include:

Managing the intake of energy - When we expend less vitality (i.e., calories) than we consume, we shed more body fat pounds. So, your consumption of energy giving food by eating smaller meals or slightly larger meals is dependent upon you.

Maintaining food quality - Crisp, natural, supplement food is an obvious requirement, paying little heed to which eating style you choose.

Cardiovascular activity (Exercise) - As we already know, to maintain perfect body shape and steady heart rate, there it is mandatory to exercise.

If you practice frequently, you require a more significant number of calories and supplements than somebody who doesn't. Your body will request those supplements by making you hungrier. If conventions intended for non-exercisers will likely influence you to feel terrible.

Obviously, non-exercisers, be careful with a similar thing. Even better, begin working out!

CHAPTER THREE

SUBJECT AND VARIETIES

According to the Canadian Medical Association Journal communicated it states that there is limited time material for the eating regimen portrayed by individuals eating unhealthy nourishment, for example, burgers, pizzas and chips, and this could energize overeating.

Psychologist the "eating window;" extend the "fasting window."

With most conventions, you map out your typical sudden fast for a predetermined timeframe – whether it's 16, 24, or 36 hours.

In like manner, you limit your typical feeding window to 4, 8, or 12 hours.

Parity focal points and disservices

Most people trust that the more extended the fast – up to yet not more than 36 hours – the more remarkable it is regarding wellbeing and sickness counteractive action benefits.

Nonetheless, longer fasts are of twofold. Choosing – and saving – lean mass is an essential fragment of healthy living and solid budding, and in the long run looking tremendous and being fit. Tragically, engaging in longer fasts pose a problem to muscle comfort and dynamism. They may likewise adversely influence the intake of supplements: Disastrously, it is almost impossible for you to have the necessary nutrients expected in a balanced diet such as vitamins, minerals, proteins, and beneficial phytonutrients.

Little wonder why health and fitness cognizant people tend to favor shorter fasts (within 15-20 hours for each day) in finally include exercises, then supplement it with an eating period of 4-9 hours. In spite of the fact that it's for the most part theory, there are two proposed benefits:

The fasting exercise can animate a physiological state like an expanded fast.

Eating more of energy supplements in the post-practice window can help with muscle recuperation and supplement dividends.

CHAPTER FOUR

EXPLORING THE BENEFITS OF INTERMITTENT FASTING

From the very time, you had your last meal until the next day mealtime (aside from the sleep cycle) makes up your "fasting" interim. Furthermore, the time from your first food of the day until the point when your last supper makes up your "feeding" interim.

Put in basic terms, if you regularly have supper by 9 PM and breakfast at 9 AM the following day, you're fasting for 12 hours long and feeding for 12 hours. A few people allude to this as a half-day fast. Although it's bizarre to give entangled names and numbers to typical examples of sleeping and eating times, yet, these will prove to be useful in a moment.

Merging Science and History together

Intermittent fasting is just the same old being brand new. People have fasted more in a lot of their history either knowingly and unknowingly, regardless of whether it's amid the regular overnight period, amid more expanded times when they come short of food, or for religious reasons.

What is new is that clinical research one's advantages for health and lifespan are starting to make up for lost time.

As earlier pointed out, intermittent fasting, when done reasonably, may help broaden lifespan, manipulate blood glucose, control blood lipids, oversee body weight, pick up (or keep up) slender mass, and many more.

Instead of something we're compelled to continue – a consequence of reduced nourishment accessibility or social desires – is getting to be something that comfort and fitness analysts are searching out with the aim of keeping their bodies fit as much as they can.

Disadvantages of intermittent fasting

• Blood lipids (counting diminished triglycerides and LDL cholesterol)

• Pulse (maybe through changes in thoughtful/parasympathetic action)

• Causes irritation (counting CRP<, IL-6, TNF, BDNF, and that's just the beginning)

• Oxidative pressure (making use of the source of protein, lipid, and keeping the DNA in danger)

Advantages

Having a quick recall of what we discussed in chapter one, fasting is essential among religious conventions for a long time now, while the medical benefits of intermittent fasting have been acknowledged since the 1940s.

However, should you in any way try to forfeit the idea of eating "three square meals per day" and try out intermittent fasting, then you'll be sure to do well to your health.

Amid times of fasting, the nerve cell circuits are more dynamic. This reason, however, is not far-fetched as there is a relationship with an increase in creating proteins in the body system called neurotrophic factors. This further proves that intermittent fasting upgrades the capacity of nerve cells to adapt to pressure and oppose against maladies as well as providing advances for clearing metabolic wastes, and diminishes aggravation as well as making necessary repair to the DNA

Potential Health Benefits

Individuals who have experienced intermittent fasting believe that there are very much advantages attached to eating regimen; some of which include:

Increased Lifespan

Some researchers have connected intermittent fasting as a means of having a more extended, and more fortifying life.

Various researchers, however, have considered the systems behind those advantages and their elucidation to people.

Let's consider this; Insulin-like development factor-1 (IGF-1) is a hormone present in the body which is connected to unambiguous maladies that influence le expectancy such as diabetes. And since most of what we devour as food contains large sequences of IGF-1, fasting might be the best approach to diminish IGF-1 levels, thereby cutting down the rate of sickness and death rates.

Tumor/Cancer

Over the years, the human race has experienced more maladies than it has ever since its existence. This is due to the immense effect of civilization and the significant effects it has on humanity. Lots of researchers have been carried out and it has proven that confining calories diminishes IGF-1 levels, which brings about a sizeable cut in the growth of the cancerous tumor and the basic strategy that brings about the development is no-farther than intermittent fasting. Fasting diminishes a substantial part of the reactions to chemotherapy.

However, due to some of the unconstructive impact, longtime calorie confinement isn't prescribed for individuals with malignancy. On the other hand, since there is still need for calorie limitation, then, intermittent fasting might be the power solution for this.

Medical analysts also claim that intermittent fasting decreases the possibility of having breast cancer.

Other advantages include;

Cell refurbishing or repair (usually referred to as autophagocytosis)

Burning off excess fats (increment in unsaturated fat deterioration later in the fast)

Development hormone discharge during fast (hormonally interceded)

Late metabolic rate during the fast (invigorated by the discharge of epinephrine and norepinephrine)

Craving control (maybe in the course of adjustments in ghrelin and PPY)

Managing glucose intake (by bringing down blood sugar and expanding insulin affectability)

Cardiovascular capacity (by offering assurance against ischemic heart damage)

Adequacy of chemotherapy (Considering higher measurements all the more regularly)

Neuronal and neuro-genesis pliancy (by providing security against neurotoxins)

With these advantages outlined, intermittent fasting has all the earmarks of being an astonishing solution. So then, why isn't everybody doing it?

Everybody is doing it, yes, everybody is doing it! Most times, individuals are fasting for virtually 12 hours daily. Unless you're an avid sleeper and wakes up only during the evening while battering the ice chest, you're most likely to get a charge out of a portion of the advantages of intermittent fasting. You simply didn't haven't noticed it or familiarize yourself with it.

Nonetheless, with regards to relative momentum, some of these advantages may just be acknowledged after longer times of fasting, contingent upon your metabolic levels. For instance, in case you're indisputably in one place amid the fast, you may require the full 20-24 hours without food or any form of nourishment to comprehend the advantages. Be that as it may, in case you're exceptionally dynamic, or you practice deliberately amid the period of your fast, you might have the capacity to appreciate similar advantages after just 16-20 hours without food.

Notice: It is emphatically suggested that you take after an activity program paying little heed to whether you're exploring different avenues regarding intermittent fasting.

Results for intermittent fasting look convincing. Considering things with the way they are, shouldn't you try it out at least to test the efficiency? Perhaps, or perhaps not. Sometimes these options looks can be confusing.

- The majority of the exploration to date has been finished utilizing creature models.

Despite the fact that creatures (like rats and monkeys) are advantageous guineas pigs, they're not ideal models for anticipating human reaction designs. Thus, all the creature information proposing substantial advantages with aren't useful in predicting what will happen when people attempt it.

When we look to the human information, we find – disappointingly – that examinations utilizing are exceptionally restricted. Additionally, those tests that have frequently been done use poor test control gatherings.

This makes their unmistakable and prescient power constrained.

(There are some brilliant surveys on this, and I'll point to them in the assets segment if you're intrigued.)

I know this is irritating. I wish science were done flawlessly inevitably, as well. Be that as it may, at present, given the available research, we're left with much a more significant number of inquiries regarding than answers. Nothing is authoritative.

As a side note, none of this is shocking. Human subjects are famously difficult to enroll for consideration into ventures, unless they're generously compensated, particularly for ventures that appear to be awkward or awkward.

Considering intermittent fasting, if you have a one-two punch. To start with, sporadic fasting thoughts don't sound all that alluring. Secondly, there aren't some massive multi-billion dollars organizations arranging to finance consideration that help to fast.

• Intermittent fasting is regularly contrasted with "typical" eating.

Regardless of whether that is standard rodent chow (on account of our fuzzy little companions) or the North American eating regimen, none of the said diets is best for comfort, body structure, or execution. In contrasting this very study, individuals utilizing intermittent fasting procedures with those using imperfect intake of nourishment without fasting, are indeed "stacking the deck" for intermittent fasting.

How? To begin with, the standard North American eating routine is regularly hyper-vivacious – they eat more than they give out– which prompts the immense cause for overweight after some time. Since intermittent fasting conventions frequently prompt a negative vitality balance – that is, we shed more pounds of fats than we take in similar to a test for both under-eating and over-eating.

Almost all controlled calorie contemplates – not only the intermittent fasting ones – showcase enhancements in a wide range of comfort and bodybuilders experts/analyst, mainly when body weight and muscle is lesser than the fat ratio in the body system.

So perhaps it's not the intermittent fasting convention that is prompting every one of the advantages discussed previously.

Maybe it's simply consuming more than we eat that has a significant effect.

Uncertain... but quite intriguing

Without the ability to control calorie intake, the typical North American eating routine is loaded with profound handled macronutrients, and added substances, laced with unknown natural poisons. By inquiring as to whether concentrates to go without nourishment for expanded periods, maybe we're not just deceiving them into eating fewer calories, we're likewise restricting their food intake of health corrupting elements.

Apparently, you may contend, that is one of the primary purposes of fasting. Be that as it may, isn't required to diminish our admission of prepared food, added substances, and poisons. Perhaps we could merely quit eating half-cooked foods, added materials, and contaminations and experience similar advantages.

Past this hypothesis, there are various reasons why the -related research is uncertain. Be that as it may, it would best not to stall this book with an excess of activity and nutritious science.

At last, I'm not endeavoring to contend for or against the advantages of intermittent fasting. It is presumed to be a cool way to deal with explaining a couple of health and body management system related issues. While sporadic fasting results look encouraging, this particular area hasn't yet advanced to the point where we can state with assurance that the advantages come only from fasting.

At present, it's similarly conceivable that:

Eating fewer calories than you consume; and

Following an eating routine lower in processed nourishments, chemicals, and contaminations

... Intermittent fasting may offer a significant portion of indistinguishable advantages of losing excess body fats. It would be nice to include a decent exercise program, and you may have the capacity to coordinate benefits for a perfect edge.

Is it the fasting or is it the negative vitality balance?

"Over 99% of the learner fat loss customers at most exercise center come there with empty stomachs, probably skipping breakfast. They don't eat between the periods of their exercises consistently. So they wind up fast in the vicinity of 16 and 18 hours most days, much the same as a great deal of the fasting campaigners suggests. Without a doubt, their dieting plans aren't grand, to begin with. However, they're fasting and not getting more slender. A considerable lot of them are increasing fat.

"When we include a solid breakfast within the 15 minutes of awakening, we see huge differences immediately. I don't know whether having breakfast causes them control hunger, prompting fewer aggregate calories eaten later in the day. I'm not totally beyond any doubt. Perhaps there are other metabolic or wholesome contrasts that assistance here as well. All I know is that ceasing the fast before anything else commences a large group of positive changes for these customers. It works without fail." Apparently, a couple of things change all the while. These customers begin practicing frequently, and this always has a significant effect. They likewise start eating an additional meal daily (most times breakfast). Those are the immediate changes.

By implication, it was figured out that including breakfast influenced meals later in the day, making them eat less. As a result of them eating breakfast, they simply weren't as eager to eat lunch or supper.

Most bodybuilding experts often wager their new sense of duty regarding comfort for these customers doesn't just drive them to hit the gym and begin having breakfast, although they do have a kind of change the kinds of food they ate, regardless of whether they weren't advised unequivocally to do as such.

That is the reason presumed by most gym instructing customers' advantage from not fasting. The whole of their two principal changes (including exercise and including a substantial breakfast) and their two auxiliary changes (enhancing food consumption and sum later in the day) prompted the most vital necessity for loss of weight: which has an adverse effect on energy balance.

Their energy usage started to surpass calories eaten. They shed lots of body pounds, get more advantageous, and enhanced their lives by fasting.

In any case, this isn't a contention for or against breakfast (or fasting). It is speculated that all else is equivalent – a not too lousy measure of activity, controlled aggregate calorie consumption, appropriate food choice, and legitimate dinner timing – it doesn't make a difference all that much whether customers have a light breakfast or skip breakfast (a far more engaging fast).

There's just a single issue: it's challenging to ensure all equation concerning fasting is balanced.

Exercise and eating choices don't work as one. One decision impacts the following, et cetera. This occurs on both the cognizant and oblivious level. What's more, there's a fascinating cross-talk between the body (physiology) and the cerebrum (mentality or psychologically).

In this manner, individuals skipping breakfast without an arrangement more often than not indulge in eating solid food later in the day. Evening over-eating is one of the most depressing issues for most people seeking to lose fat as well. These outcomes are pre-arranged in more muscle versus fat, exposing them to a higher danger of diabetes, and a broader group of other medical issues. That is why most medical analysts prescribe that individuals new to eating admirably and practicing should start from having breakfast, as time goes on, they can begin skipping meals – although they must have a well-structured plan to follow.

On a more important notice: It's not the breakfast that matters, but rather what comes after the breakfast that is far more important.

Be that as it may, it appears like the individuals who have a decent arrangement for controlling calories later in the day and stays with it can escape with skipping breakfast with no adverse results.

So indeed, breakfast might be a passing time when you've correctly figured out how best to monitor your eating choices for the whole day.

That is the reason self-experimentation and way of life coordinating are exceptionally fundamental. If you need to boost your results, you'll need to make sense of how you react to having breakfast or skipping it. Things like marking out essential dates in your calendar, your unique physiology, and your self-restraint will assume a significant part here.

As the look into intermittent fasting program proceeds, we'll be observing intently to perceive what happens when calorie-controlled, supplement thick, and stable diets are contrasted with calorie-controlled, supplement compact, healthy weight loss design that doesn't utilize expanded fasts. Until these investigations are complete, only then can we truly know whether the enchantment is in the – or out of enhancing food sum and nourishment choice.

That examination could take quite a while, however. This is my sincere recommendation: Don't hold up until the point when these investigations are ascertained to be true. Control your intake of food and always for quantity. Also, try starting up an activity program if possible immediately, and as time goes on, you'll get many, if not all, of the advantages above.

Apparently, it is easier to say than to act. Medical/health experts always advise individuals to "eat less and exercise more." Most times, that method hasn't been working so well.

You should attempt further developed conventions like intermittent fasting after you've manufactured this strong making. Probably a one-time, one-day fast, as proposed in the presentation wouldn't be such a bad idea.

Much the same as the popular thought in high school, you need to take in and understand the rules first before you can break them. Conclusively, a person who's been practicing and eating great for almost 20 years – has aced the fundamentals.

However, it's time to break a few rules.

CONCLUSION

Thank you again for purchasing this book! I hope it was able to help you learn how to apply the practice of Intermittent Fasting in your le's schedules to reap the immense benefits inherent in it and so, become a healthier, happier, better, and yes, wealthier you.

The next step is to put all you have learned into practice and watch your le shine!

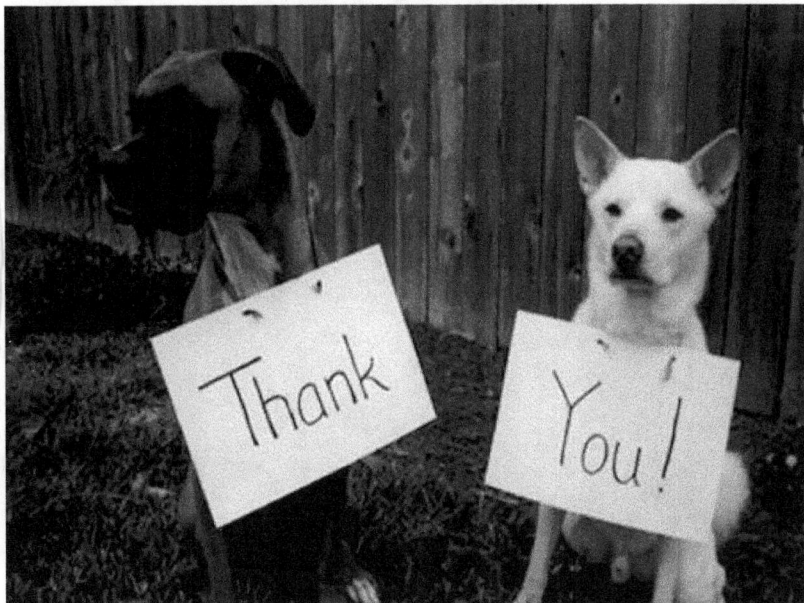

Finally, you enjoyed this book; then I'd like to ask you for a favor; would you be kind enough to leave a review for this book? It'd be much appreciated!

Thank you and good luck!

www.ingramcontent.com/pod-product-compliance
Lightning Source LLC
Chambersburg PA
CBHW070258290326
41930CB00041B/2647